My Child's Food Allergy Diary

A 45-day diary to find your child's food allergies for a healthy life

Ceri Clark

My Child's Food Allergy Diary: A 45-day diary to find your child's food allergies for a healthy life

© 2017 Cover & Interior Design: Ceri Clark

First Edition
ISBN-10: 1544140894
ISBN-13: 978-1544140896
Published by
Myrddin Publishing Group
Contact us at - www.myrddinpublishing.com

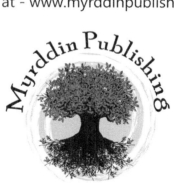

unique electronic & print books

Name

Known Allergies

Illnesses

Current Medication

You must always consult your doctor in the first instance and in most cases they will suggest you track your child's eating habits. This book is designed to help you do this.

Why I created this book

I created this book to see if my son was allergic to anything. I am allergic to quite a few foods and I wanted to see if a few problems he was experiencing were down to food. I had to create this for myself so I thought rather than keeping it in a drawer I should share it with the world!

A word of warning

Do not use this book to test for foods where you know your child already has an

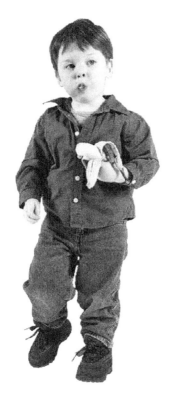

INTRODUCTION

Allergies can range from the mildly annoying to the horrific. What we can be allergic to can be as diverse as the symptoms we suffer.

Filling out this journal can help you to find out patterns which will help you pinpoint any allergies your child may have developed.

allergy. Reactions can be dangerous and you should always go for allergy testing with a medical professional.

Over use of an allergic substance can make an allergy worse. For example I tested allergic to citrus fruits as a child but only mildly allergic. I didn't realise that the allergy could get worse if I consumed a large quantity of citrus fruits. While I was at university, I drank 2 large bottles of fizzy lemonade. Let's just say I really reacted and ever since I cannot tolerate any citrus, not even citric acid. If I had known then what I know now I'd be shrieking at my former self not to drink it! Oh well, we live and learn.

How to fill out the day-by-day information

Food and drink

Always put in how much of something they eat, eg 1 banana, 2 chocolate chip cookies. If you can, list the ingredients from the packet. Everyone has busy lives so this may not always be possible. There is a quick checkbox list at the bottom of the page of common allergens to save you time on those busy days.

Drinks

It is easy to forget drinks but drinking water can really help with symptoms such as eczema or constipation. Other drinks can contain hidden allergens. If you know that your child reacts when he or she drinks something then you can go back and look at the ingredients later.

Common allergy triggers

These are checkboxes for the most common triggers of allergies. This is to save you time when you are looking at your results. The most common triggers include dairy, soy (soya in the UK), eggs, gluten, nuts, fruit, shellfish, and fish. At the end of this section there are 'cards' which set out the main foods to look out for which contain these ingredients.

Filling out these boxes will really help you and your doctor when scanning through the pages when the book is complete.

How many drinks has your child had?

The NHS (The National Health Service in the UK) website states that 6-8 glasses of fluid a day should be drunk each day. Surprisingly, this can include water, drinks that can contain caffeine (e.g. soft drinks and hot chocolate, not just tea or coffee) and milk.

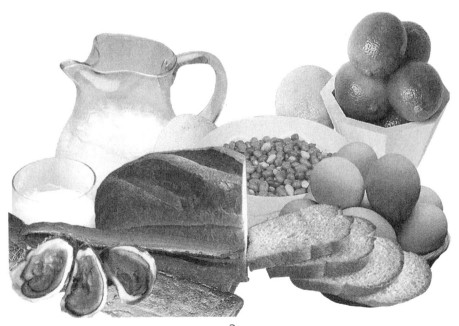

Milk is important for young children as it contains calcium and important vitamins. However, if your child is allergic to dairy products then there are now some good alternatives. As long as you watch the calories and caffeine in drinks, you can make healthy choices.

Keep track of how many drinks your child has in the box next to the picture of the glass.

How is your child feeling?

Are they sad, feeling okay or really happy today? Tick, cross or circle the smiley that best reflects your child's mood.

Symptoms

Are they more tired than usual, are their lips swelling or is there an itch that just won't go away? How bad are the symptoms compared to the day before? Are they feeling better?

Colds, flu and other bugs

Those nasty critters which make us unwell when we least expect it can affect other conditions. Tick the box beside cold, flu and stomach bugs to help explain why your child might be unwell even though there is no food or drink eaten or drunk which could explain it.

Stools

It can be embarrassing talking about our, ahem, waste but luckily for the more shy among us, the medical profession have come up with the *Bristol Stool Chart*. Rather than describing in excrutiating detail what comes out of our derrière we can just say number 4 with a smile on our faces. It may sound like you are ordering a takeaway but if it saves my blushes I'm all for it.

Please take a look at the chart on the next page for a quick reference to how healthy your child's poop is!

Bristol Stool Chart

 Type 1 Separate hard lumps

 Type 2 Lumpy and sausage like

 Type 3 A sausage shape with cracks in the surface

 Type 4 Like a smooth, soft sausage or snake

 Type 5 Soft blobs with clear-cut edges

 Type 6 Mushy consistency with ragged edges

 Type 7 Liquid consistency with no solid pieces

The chart above is adapted from a Photo by Cabot Health, Bristol Stool Chart / CC BY SA (available from Wikimedia)

Each child is different so you are looking for changes but types 3-5 are in the normal range.

Comments

The comments section on the diary pages are for anything not covered in the other boxes. This can include medication and any chronic conditions your child may have.

The summary table

At the back of this book there is a summary table. Fill in the foods, whether an illness has developed or if the stools are less than ideal in the days that are applicable to get a quick overview to spot trends easily.

You can fill as much or as little of this book as you want to but the more you fill in the more data your doctor will have to work out what is affecting your child. The next page gives an example of how the diary pages can be filled out.

Example diary pages filled out.

How are you today? 🙂 😐 😊 [6]

Time	Food and Drink
8.00	1 glass of milk, 2 toast with butter
9.00	1 glass of apple juice
11.00	Chocolate bar
1.00	Ham sandwich with butter — white bread.
2.30	Handful of peanuts
5.30	Burger and fries

Time	Symptoms
8.30	arms red e itchy
3.00	lips tingly.

COMMON ALLERGY TRIGGERS

☐ Celery
☑ Dairy
☐ Eggs
☐ Fish
☑ Fruit
☑ Gluten
☐ Lupin(e)
☐ Mustard
☑ Nuts
☐ Sesame Seeds
☐ Sulphites
☐ Shellfish
☐ Soy(a)

Do you have a cold/flu or stomach bug? ☐ Yes ☑ No

Stools ❶ ❷ ❸ ❹ ⑤ ❻ ❼
See page 5 for scale
Hard   Normal range   Liquid

Comments

Summary table

Common Triggers	1	2	3	4	5	6	7	8	9	10	11
Any reaction?	✓										
Dairy	✓										
Soy(a)											
Eggs											
Nuts	✓										
Fruit	✓										
Shellfish											
Fish											
Illness											
Stools (1-7)	5										
Other											

Celery

Batter for frozen foods
Canned soups
Celery leaves

Celery seeds, which are sometimes used to make celery salt
Celery spice
Celery sticks
Crisps
Marmite

Pre-prepared sandwiches
Salads
Spice mixes
Stock cubes

Dairy

Butter
Butter fat
Butter flavoring ghee
Butter oil
Buttermilk
Cakes
Calcium casein
Casein
Casein

hydrolysate
Cheese
Crème fraiche
Dark chocolate**
Fromage frais
Ice cream
Lactaglobulin, lactose
Lactalbumin
Lactoalbumin phosphate
Lactoferrin
Lactulose
Magenesium

casein
Non-dairy creamers
Olive Spread
Potassium casein
Rennet casein
Pudding, sour cream
Sodium casein
Whey
Whey hydrolysate
Yoghurt

This list only contains the most common foods that these allergens appear in. Please check the labels of everything your child eats as these ingredients can be added to any food without warning.

**Some dark chocolate may not contain dairy.*

7

Eggs

Biscuits
Boiled egg
Bread & butter pudding
Breadcrumbs
Cakes
Cheeses
Chocolate bars with fillings
Dried egg noodles
Dried egg pasta
Egg fried rice
Egg glaze on pastry
Egg in batter
Egg pasta
Flan
Fresh Mousse
Fried egg
Gravy granules
Hollandaise sauce
Horseradish sauce
Ice creams
Lemon curd
Marzipan
Mayonnaise
Meringues
Omelette
Pancakes
Poached egg
Quiche
Quorn
Raw egg in cake mix and other similar dishes before cooking
Royal icing (fresh and powdered royal icing sugar)
Salad cream
Scotch egg
Scotch pancakes
Scrambled egg
Sorbets
Spanish tortilla
Tartare sauce
Tempura batter
Waffles
Yorkshire puddings

Fish

Anchovy
Basa
Bouillabaisse
Cod
Cuttlefish
Eel
Etouffee
Flounder
Fritto Misto
Grouper
Gumbo
Haddock
Hake
Halibut
Jambalaya
Kedgeree
Mackerel
Monkfish
Perch
Pike
Pilchards
Plaice
Pollock
Salmon
Sardine
Sea bass
Sea bream
Snapper
Swordfish
Trout
Tuna
Turbot
Whitebait
Whiting

Fruit

Any fruits can beome an allergen including but not limited to:

Citrus fruits (oranges, lemons etc.)

Raspberries

Tomatoes

Gluten

Ale

Beer

Bread and baked foods

Burgers

Cakes and deserts with a biscuit base

Candy (Sweets)

Cereals

Chocolate

Chocolate bars

Chocolate drinks

Continental sausages

Corned beef

Fish

Fish pastes and spreads

Flour and pasta

Gin

Ham

Ice cream

Larger

Liquorice

Liver-sausage

Luncheon meat

Malted milk

Meat

Meat and Fish covered in breadcrumbs

Ovaltine

Pancakes

Pastry

Pates

Puddings

Rissoles

Salami

Sauces and condiments

Sausages

Scotch eggs

Soups

Spirits

Stout

Tinned beans

Vegetables coated in breadcrumbs (onion rings)

Vegetables tempura

Yogurts containing cereal

Lupin(e) Crepe	Deep-coated vegetables such as onion rings Lupin Flour Pancakes	Pastry cases Pies Pizzas Waffles
Mustard	Deli meats (the coating) Pickled onions Sauces including	mayonaisse and salad dressings Table mustards
Nuts Biscuits Cakes Cereal bars Confectionery	Curries and other Eastern dishes Desserts Ice cream Marzipan Pastries Peanut shoots (they look like	bean sprouts) Pesto sauce Praline Salad dressings Salads Satay sauce Vegetarian products
Sesame Seeds Aqua Libra (a drink) Biscuits Bread	Breadsticks Chinese stir-fry oils (sesame oil) Crackers Burger buns Furikake (a seasoning) Gomashio Halvah	health food snacks Hummus Salad dishes Stir-fry vegetables Tahini Vegeburgers
Sulphites Coconut milk Dehydrated vegetables like dried onions Dehydrated,	pre-cut or peeled potatoes Dried fruits and vegetables Fresh or frozen prawns Frozen and raw potato products Fruits sprayed	with sulphites including apricots, grapes and sultanas

Shellfish		
	Crayfish	Prawns
	Lobster	Scallop
	Shrimp	Scampi
Abalone	Mussel	Snail
Clam	Octopus	Squid (calamari)
Cockle	Oyster	Whelks
Crab	Periwinkle	

Soy(a)		
	Cakes	(E322)
	Biscuits	Soy sauce
	Infant foods	
Tofu (soya bean curd	Vegetable protein	
Bread	Soya lecithin	

Please note there are other allergens which are not classed as food which have not been covered by this book which include for example, ingredients in medication (always check the leaflets) and other allergens such as latex (rubber), perfume and pollen.

Always read the labels on food and consult your doctor when testing for allergies. This is only one tool in the toolbox to help you identify allergies. There are so many factors that could lead to a reaction, some of which can lead to an instant reaction and others accumulative, from what we eat, drink, touch and breath.

The best way to avoid allergic reactions is to avoid the substances that cause a reaction in the first place. This book aims to help you to sort out food and drink which are the easiest allergens to avoid.

DIARY
PAGES

Day 1

Time	Food and Drink

COMMON ALLERGY TRIGGERS

❑ Celery
❑ Dairy
❑ Eggs
❑ Fish
❑ Fruit
❑ Gluten
❑ Lupin(e)

❑ Mustard
❑ Nuts
❑ Sesame Seeds
❑ Sulphites
❑ Shellfish
❑ Soy(a)

14

	How are you today?
Time	Symptons

Do you have a cold/flu or stomach bug? ☐ Yes ☐ No

Stools
See page 5 for scale
❶ ❷ ❸ ❹ ❺ ❻ ❼
Hard   Normal range   Liquid

Comments

Day 2

Time	Food and Drink

COMMON ALLERGY TRIGGERS

❑ Celery
❑ Dairy
❑ Eggs
❑ Fish
❑ Fruit
❑ Gluten
❑ Lupin(e)

❑ Mustard
❑ Nuts
❑ Sesame Seeds
❑ Sulphites
❑ Shellfish
❑ Soy(a)

How are you today?

Time	Symptons

Do you have a cold/flu or stomach bug? ❏ Yes ❏ No

Stools
See page 5 for scale

❶ ❷ ❸ ❹ ❺ ❻ ❼

Hard   Normal range   Liquid

Comments

Day 3

Time	Food and Drink

COMMON ALLERGY TRIGGERS

❑ Celery
❑ Dairy
❑ Eggs
❑ Fish
❑ Fruit
❑ Gluten
❑ Lupin(e)

❑ Mustard
❑ Nuts
❑ Sesame Seeds
❑ Sulphites
❑ Shellfish
❑ Soy(a)

18

How are you today?

Time	Symptons

Do you have a cold/flu or stomach bug? ❑ Yes ❑ No

Stools
See page 5 for scale

❶ ❷ ❸ ❹ ❺ ❻ ❼

Hard   Normal range   Liquid

Comments

Day 4

Time	Food and Drink

COMMON ALLERGY TRIGGERS

- ❑ Celery
- ❑ Dairy
- ❑ Eggs
- ❑ Fish
- ❑ Fruit
- ❑ Gluten
- ❑ Lupin(e)

- ❑ Mustard
- ❑ Nuts
- ❑ Sesame Seeds
- ❑ Sulphites
- ❑ Shellfish
- ❑ Soy(a)

20

How are you today?

Time	Symptons

Do you have a cold/flu or stomach bug? ❑ Yes ❑ No

Stools
See page 5 for scale

❶   ❷   ❸   ❹   ❺   ❻   ❼

Hard   Normal range   Liquid

Comments

Day 5

Time	Food and Drink

COMMON ALLERGY TRIGGERS

❑ Celery
❑ Dairy
❑ Eggs
❑ Fish
❑ Fruit
❑ Gluten
❑ Lupin(e)

❑ Mustard
❑ Nuts
❑ Sesame Seeds
❑ Sulphites
❑ Shellfish
❑ Soy(a)

22

How are you today?

Time	Symptons

Do you have a cold/flu or stomach bug? ❑ Yes ❑ No

Stools
See page 5 for scale

❶ ❷ ❸ ❹ ❺ ❻ ❼

Hard   Normal range   Liquid

Comments

Day 6

Time	Food and Drink

COMMON ALLERGY TRIGGERS

❑ Celery
❑ Dairy
❑ Eggs
❑ Fish
❑ Fruit
❑ Gluten
❑ Lupin(e)

❑ Mustard
❑ Nuts
❑ Sesame Seeds
❑ Sulphites
❑ Shellfish
❑ Soy(a)

24

How are you today?

Time	Symptons

Do you have a cold/flu or stomach bug? ❑ Yes ❑ No

Stools
See page 5 for scale

❶ ❷ ❸ ❹ ❺ ❻ ❼

Hard   Normal range   Liquid

Comments

Day 7

Time	Food and Drink

COMMON ALLERGY TRIGGERS

❑ Celery
❑ Dairy
❑ Eggs
❑ Fish
❑ Fruit
❑ Gluten
❑ Lupin(e)

❑ Mustard
❑ Nuts
❑ Sesame Seeds
❑ Sulphites
❑ Shellfish
❑ Soy(a)

26

How are you today?

Time	Symptons

Do you have a cold/flu or stomach bug? ❑ Yes ❑ No

Stools
See page 5 for scale

❶ ❷ ❸ ❹ ❺ ❻ ❼

Hard　　　Normal range　　　Liquid

Comments

Day 8

Time	Food and Drink

COMMON ALLERGY TRIGGERS

- ❏ Celery
- ❏ Dairy
- ❏ Eggs
- ❏ Fish
- ❏ Fruit
- ❏ Gluten
- ❏ Lupin(e)

- ❏ Mustard
- ❏ Nuts
- ❏ Sesame Seeds
- ❏ Sulphites
- ❏ Shellfish
- ❏ Soy(a)

☐ *How are you today?*

Time	Symptons

Do you have a cold/flu or stomach bug? ☐ Yes ☐ No

Stools
See page 5 for scale

❶ ❷ ❸ ❹ ❺ ❻ ❼

Hard   Normal range   Liquid

Comments

Day 9

Time	Food and Drink

COMMON ALLERGY TRIGGERS

❑ Celery
❑ Dairy
❑ Eggs
❑ Fish
❑ Fruit
❑ Gluten
❑ Lupin(e)

❑ Mustard
❑ Nuts
❑ Sesame Seeds
❑ Sulphites
❑ Shellfish
❑ Soy(a)

30

How are you today?

Time	Symptons

Do you have a cold/flu or stomach bug? ☐ Yes ☐ No

Stools
See page 5 for scale

❶　❷　❸　❹　❺　❻　❼

Hard　　Normal range　　Liquid

Comments

31

Day 10

Time	Food and Drink

COMMON ALLERGY TRIGGERS

- ☐ Celery
- ☐ Dairy
- ☐ Eggs
- ☐ Fish
- ☐ Fruit
- ☐ Gluten
- ☐ Lupin(e)

- ☐ Mustard
- ☐ Nuts
- ☐ Sesame Seeds
- ☐ Sulphites
- ☐ Shellfish
- ☐ Soy(a)

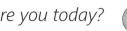 *How are you today?*

Time	Symptons

Do you have a cold/flu or stomach bug? ❑ Yes ❑ No

Stools
See page 5 for scale

❶ ❷ ❸ ❹ ❺ ❻ ❼

Hard   Normal range   Liquid

Comments

Day 11

Time	Food and Drink

- ☐ Celery
- ☐ Dairy
- ☐ Eggs
- ☐ Fish
- ☐ Fruit
- ☐ Gluten
- ☐ Lupin(e)

- ☐ Mustard
- ☐ Nuts
- ☐ Sesame Seeds
- ☐ Sulphites
- ☐ Shellfish
- ☐ Soy(a)

☐ *How are you today?*

Time	Symptons

Do you have a cold/flu or stomach bug? ☐ Yes ☐ No

Stools
See page 5 for scale

Hard · Normal range · Liquid

Comments

Day 12

Time	Food and Drink

COMMON ALLERGY TRIGGERS

- ❑ Celery
- ❑ Dairy
- ❑ Eggs
- ❑ Fish
- ❑ Fruit
- ❑ Gluten
- ❑ Lupin(e)

- ❑ Mustard
- ❑ Nuts
- ❑ Sesame Seeds
- ❑ Sulphites
- ❑ Shellfish
- ❑ Soy(a)

How are you today?

Time	Symptons

Do you have a cold/flu or stomach bug? ❑ Yes ❑ No

Stools
See page 5 for scale

① **②** **③** **④** **⑤** **⑥** **⑦**

Hard   Normal range   Liquid

Comments

Day 13

Time	Food and Drink

COMMON ALLERGY TRIGGERS

❑ Celery
❑ Dairy
❑ Eggs
❑ Fish
❑ Fruit
❑ Gluten
❑ Lupin(e)

❑ Mustard
❑ Nuts
❑ Sesame Seeds
❑ Sulphites
❑ Shellfish
❑ Soy(a)

38

How are you today?

Time	Symptons

Do you have a cold/flu or stomach bug? ❑ Yes ❑ No

Stools
See page 5 for scale

1   **2**   **3**   **4**   **5**   **6**   **7**

Hard   Normal range   Liquid

Comments

Day 14

Time	Food and Drink

COMMON ALLERGY TRIGGERS

- ❑ Celery
- ❑ Dairy
- ❑ Eggs
- ❑ Fish
- ❑ Fruit
- ❑ Gluten
- ❑ Lupin(e)

- ❑ Mustard
- ❑ Nuts
- ❑ Sesame Seeds
- ❑ Sulphites
- ❑ Shellfish
- ❑ Soy(a)

How are you today?

Time	Symptons

Do you have a cold/flu or stomach bug? ❏ Yes ❏ No

Stools
See page 5 for scale

❶ ❷ ❸ ❹ ❺ ❻ ❼

Hard   Normal range   Liquid

Comments

Day 15

Time	Food and Drink

❏ Celery
❏ Dairy
❏ Eggs
❏ Fish
❏ Fruit
❏ Gluten
❏ Lupin(e)

❏ Mustard
❏ Nuts
❏ Sesame Seeds
❏ Sulphites
❏ Shellfish
❏ Soy(a)

How are you today?

Time	Symptons

Do you have a cold/flu or stomach bug? ❑ Yes ❑ No

Stools
See page 5 for scale

❶ ❷ ❸ ❹ ❺ ❻ ❼

Hard   Normal range   Liquid

Comments

Day 16

Time	Food and Drink

How are you today?

Time	Symptons

Do you have a cold/flu or stomach bug? ❏ Yes ❏ No

Stools
See page 5 for scale

❶ ❷ ❸ ❹ ❺ ❻ ❼

Hard · Normal range · Liquid

Comments

Day 17

Time	Food and Drink

❑ Celery
❑ Dairy
❑ Eggs
❑ Fish
❑ Fruit
❑ Gluten
❑ Lupin(e)

❑ Mustard
❑ Nuts
❑ Sesame Seeds
❑ Sulphites
❑ Shellfish
❑ Soy(a)

46

☐   *How are you today?*

Time	Symptons

Do you have a cold/flu or stomach bug? ☐ Yes ☐ No

Stools   ❶   ❷   ❸   ❹   ❺   ❻   ❼
See page 5 for scale
Hard   Normal range   Liquid

Comments

Day 18

Time	Food and Drink

COMMON ALLERGY TRIGGERS

❑ Celery
❑ Dairy
❑ Eggs
❑ Fish
❑ Fruit
❑ Gluten
❑ Lupin(e)

❑ Mustard
❑ Nuts
❑ Sesame Seeds
❑ Sulphites
❑ Shellfish
❑ Soy(a)

48

How are you today?

Time	Symptons

Do you have a cold/flu or stomach bug? ❏ Yes ❏ No

Stools
See page 5 for scale

❶ **❷** **❸** **❹** **❺** **❻** **❼**

Hard   Normal range   Liquid

Comments

49

Day 19

Time	Food and Drink

How are you today?

Time	Symptons

Do you have a cold/flu or stomach bug? ❑ Yes ❑ No

Stools ❶ ❷ ❸ ❹ ❺ ❻ ❼
See page 5 for scale
Hard   Normal range   Liquid

Comments

Day 20

Time	Food and Drink

COMMON ALLERGY TRIGGERS

❑ Celery
❑ Dairy
❑ Eggs
❑ Fish
❑ Fruit
❑ Gluten
❑ Lupin(e)

❑ Mustard
❑ Nuts
❑ Sesame Seeds
❑ Sulphites
❑ Shellfish
❑ Soy(a)

52

□ *How are you today?*

Time	Symptons

Do you have a cold/flu or stomach bug? ❑ Yes ❑ No

Stools
See page 5 for scale

❶ ❷ ❸ ❹ ❺ ❻ ❼

Hard   Normal range   Liquid

Comments

Day 21

Time	Food and Drink

❑ Celery
❑ Dairy
❑ Eggs
❑ Fish
❑ Fruit
❑ Gluten
❑ Lupin(e)

❑ Mustard
❑ Nuts
❑ Sesame Seeds
❑ Sulphites
❑ Shellfish
❑ Soy(a)

☐ *How are you today?*

Time	Symptons

Do you have a cold/flu or stomach bug? ☐ Yes ☐ No

Stools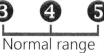
See page 5 for scale

        Hard   Normal range   Liquid

Comments

Day 22

Time	Food and Drink

COMMON ALLERGY TRIGGERS

- ❑ Celery
- ❑ Dairy
- ❑ Eggs
- ❑ Fish
- ❑ Fruit
- ❑ Gluten
- ❑ Lupin(e)

- ❑ Mustard
- ❑ Nuts
- ❑ Sesame Seeds
- ❑ Sulphites
- ❑ Shellfish
- ❑ Soy(a)

56

How are you today?

Time	Symptons

Do you have a cold/flu or stomach bug? ❑ Yes ❑ No

Stools
See page 5 for scale

❶ ❷ ❸ ❹ ❺ ❻ ❼

Hard   Normal range   Liquid

Comments

Day 23

Time	Food and Drink

COMMON ALLERGY TRIGGERS

❑ Celery
❑ Dairy
❑ Eggs
❑ Fish
❑ Fruit
❑ Gluten
❑ Lupin(e)

❑ Mustard
❑ Nuts
❑ Sesame Seeds
❑ Sulphites
❑ Shellfish
❑ Soy(a)

☐ *How are you today?*

Time	Symptons

Do you have a cold/flu or stomach bug? ☐ Yes ☐ No

Stools
See page 5 for scale

❶ ❷ ❸ ❹ ❺ ❻ ❼

Hard   Normal range   Liquid

Comments

Day 24

Time	Food and Drink

COMMON ALLERGY TRIGGERS

❑ Celery
❑ Dairy
❑ Eggs
❑ Fish
❑ Fruit
❑ Gluten
❑ Lupin(e)

❑ Mustard
❑ Nuts
❑ Sesame Seeds
❑ Sulphites
❑ Shellfish
❑ Soy(a)

60

How are you today?

Time	Symptons

Do you have a cold/flu or stomach bug? ❏ Yes ❏ No

Stools
See page 5 for scale

❶ ❷ ❸ ❹ ❺ ❻ ❼

Hard   Normal range   Liquid

Comments

Day 25

Time	Food and Drink

❏ Celery
❏ Dairy
❏ Eggs
❏ Fish
❏ Fruit
❏ Gluten
❏ Lupin(e)

❏ Mustard
❏ Nuts
❏ Sesame Seeds
❏ Sulphites
❏ Shellfish
❏ Soy(a)

How are you today?

Time	Symptons

Do you have a cold/flu or stomach bug? ❑ Yes ❑ No

Stools
See page 5 for scale

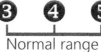

❶ ❷ ❸ ❹ ❺ ❻ ❼

Hard Normal range Liquid

Comments

Day 26

Time	Food and Drink

COMMON ALLERGY TRIGGERS

❏ Celery
❏ Dairy
❏ Eggs
❏ Fish
❏ Fruit
❏ Gluten
❏ Lupin(e)

❏ Mustard
❏ Nuts
❏ Sesame Seeds
❏ Sulphites
❏ Shellfish
❏ Soy(a)

64

How are you today?

Time	Symptons

Do you have a cold/flu or stomach bug? ❏ Yes ❏ No

Stools
See page 5 for scale

① **②** **③** **④** **⑤** **⑥** **⑦**

Hard   Normal range   Liquid

Comments

Day 27

Time	Food and Drink

❑ Celery
❑ Dairy
❑ Eggs
❑ Fish
❑ Fruit
❑ Gluten
❑ Lupin(e)

❑ Mustard
❑ Nuts
❑ Sesame Seeds
❑ Sulphites
❑ Shellfish
❑ Soy(a)

☐ *How are you today?*

Time	Symptons

Do you have a cold/flu or stomach bug? ☐ Yes ☐ No

Stools
See page 5 for scale

   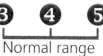

Hard   Normal range   Liquid

Comments

Day 28

Time	Food and Drink

❑ Celery
❑ Dairy
❑ Eggs
❑ Fish
❑ Fruit
❑ Gluten
❑ Lupin(e)

❑ Mustard
❑ Nuts
❑ Sesame Seeds
❑ Sulphites
❑ Shellfish
❑ Soy(a)

How are you today?

Time	Symptons

Do you have a cold/flu or stomach bug? ❑ Yes ❑ No

Stools
See page 5 for scale

❶   ❷   ❸   ❹   ❺   ❻   ❼

Hard   Normal range   Liquid

Comments

Day 29

Time	Food and Drink

COMMON ALLERGY TRIGGERS

❑ Celery
❑ Dairy
❑ Eggs
❑ Fish
❑ Fruit
❑ Gluten
❑ Lupin(e)

❑ Mustard
❑ Nuts
❑ Sesame Seeds
❑ Sulphites
❑ Shellfish
❑ Soy(a)

70

How are you today?

Time	Symptons

Do you have a cold/flu or stomach bug? ❑ Yes ❑ No

Stools
See page 5 for scale

❶ **❷** **❸** **❹** **❺** **❻** **❼**

Hard   Normal range   Liquid

Comments

Day 30

Time	Food and Drink

COMMON ALLERGY TRIGGERS

- ☐ Celery
- ☐ Dairy
- ☐ Eggs
- ☐ Fish
- ☐ Fruit
- ☐ Gluten
- ☐ Lupin(e)
- ☐ Mustard
- ☐ Nuts
- ☐ Sesame Seeds
- ☐ Sulphites
- ☐ Shellfish
- ☐ Soy(a)

72

□ _How are you today?_

Time	Symptons

Do you have a cold/flu or stomach bug? ❏ Yes ❏ No

Stools ❶ ❷ ❸ ❹ ❺ ❻ ❼
See page 5 for scale
          Hard   Normal range   Liquid

Comments

Day 31

Time	Food and Drink

❑ Celery
❑ Dairy
❑ Eggs
❑ Fish
❑ Fruit
❑ Gluten
❑ Lupin(e)

❑ Mustard
❑ Nuts
❑ Sesame Seeds
❑ Sulphites
❑ Shellfish
❑ Soy(a)

How are you today?

Time	Symptons

Do you have a cold/flu or stomach bug? ❏ Yes ❏ No

Stools
See page 5 for scale

Hard   Normal range   Liquid

Comments

Day 32

Time	Food and Drink

❑ Celery
❑ Dairy
❑ Eggs
❑ Fish
❑ Fruit
❑ Gluten
❑ Lupin(e)

❑ Mustard
❑ Nuts
❑ Sesame Seeds
❑ Sulphites
❑ Shellfish
❑ Soy(a)

☐ *How are you today?*

Time	Symptons

Do you have a cold/flu or stomach bug? ☐ Yes ☐ No

Stools
See page 5 for scale

Hard   Normal range   Liquid

Comments

Day 33

Time	Food and Drink

COMMON
ALLERGY TRIGGERS

❑ Celery
❑ Dairy
❑ Eggs
❑ Fish
❑ Fruit
❑ Gluten
❑ Lupin(e)

❑ Mustard
❑ Nuts
❑ Sesame Seeds
❑ Sulphites
❑ Shellfish
❑ Soy(a)

78

How are you today?

Time	Symptons

Do you have a cold/flu or stomach bug? ❑ Yes ❑ No

Stools
See page 5 for scale

Hard   Normal range   Liquid

Comments

Day 34

Time	Food and Drink

❑ Celery
❑ Dairy
❑ Eggs
❑ Fish
❑ Fruit
❑ Gluten
❑ Lupin(e)

❑ Mustard
❑ Nuts
❑ Sesame Seeds
❑ Sulphites
❑ Shellfish
❑ Soy(a)

How are you today?

Time	Symptons

Do you have a cold/flu or stomach bug? ☐ Yes ☐ No

Stools
See page 5 for scale

❶ ❷ ❸ ❹ ❺ ❻ ❼

Hard   Normal range   Liquid

Comments

Day 35

Time	Food and Drink

☐ *How are you today?*

Time	Symptons

Do you have a cold/flu or stomach bug? ☐ Yes ☐ No

Stools
See page 5 for scale

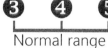

❶ ❷ ❸ ❹ ❺ ❻ ❼

Hard   Normal range   Liquid

Comments

Day 36

Time	Food and Drink

COMMON ALLERGY TRIGGERS

❑ Celery
❑ Dairy
❑ Eggs
❑ Fish
❑ Fruit
❑ Gluten
❑ Lupin(e)

❑ Mustard
❑ Nuts
❑ Sesame Seeds
❑ Sulphites
❑ Shellfish
❑ Soy(a)

84

☐ *How are you today?*

Time	Symptons

Do you have a cold/flu or stomach bug? ☐ Yes ☐ No

Stools
See page 5 for scale

❶   **❷**   **❸**   **❹**   **❺**   **❻**   **❼**

Hard   Normal range   Liquid

Comments

Day 37

Time	Food and Drink

COMMON ALLERGY TRIGGERS

❑ Celery
❑ Dairy
❑ Eggs
❑ Fish
❑ Fruit
❑ Gluten
❑ Lupin(e)

❑ Mustard
❑ Nuts
❑ Sesame Seeds
❑ Sulphites
❑ Shellfish
❑ Soy(a)

86

How are you today?

Time	Symptons

Do you have a cold/flu or stomach bug? ❑ Yes ❑ No

Stools   ❶   ❷   ❸   ❹   ❺   ❻   ❼
See page 5 for scale
                Hard   Normal range   Liquid

Comments

Day 38

Time	Food and Drink

COMMON ALLERGY TRIGGERS

❑ Celery
❑ Dairy
❑ Eggs
❑ Fish
❑ Fruit
❑ Gluten
❑ Lupin(e)

❑ Mustard
❑ Nuts
❑ Sesame Seeds
❑ Sulphites
❑ Shellfish
❑ Soy(a)

88

How are you today?

Time	Symptons

Do you have a cold/flu or stomach bug? ❑ Yes ❑ No

Stools   ❶   ❷   ❸   ❹   ❺   ❻   ❼
See page 5 for scale
          Hard   Normal range   Liquid

Comments

89

Day 39

Time	Food and Drink

COMMON ALLERGY TRIGGERS

- ☐ Celery
- ☐ Dairy
- ☐ Eggs
- ☐ Fish
- ☐ Fruit
- ☐ Gluten
- ☐ Lupin(e)

- ☐ Mustard
- ☐ Nuts
- ☐ Sesame Seeds
- ☐ Sulphites
- ☐ Shellfish
- ☐ Soy(a)

How are you today?

Time	Symptons

Do you have a cold/flu or stomach bug? ❑ Yes ❑ No

Stools
See page 5 for scale

  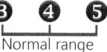

Hard   Normal range   Liquid

Comments

Day 40

Time	Food and Drink

COMMON ALLERGY TRIGGERS

❏ Celery
❏ Dairy
❏ Eggs
❏ Fish
❏ Fruit
❏ Gluten
❏ Lupin(e)

❏ Mustard
❏ Nuts
❏ Sesame Seeds
❏ Sulphites
❏ Shellfish
❏ Soy(a)

92

How are you today?

Time	Symptons

Do you have a cold/flu or stomach bug? ❏ Yes ❏ No

Stools
See page 5 for scale

Hard   Normal range   Liquid

Comments

Day 41

Time	Food and Drink

COMMON ALLERGY TRIGGERS

❑ Celery
❑ Dairy
❑ Eggs
❑ Fish
❑ Fruit
❑ Gluten
❑ Lupin(e)

❑ Mustard
❑ Nuts
❑ Sesame Seeds
❑ Sulphites
❑ Shellfish
❑ Soy(a)

94

□ *How are you today?*

Time	Symptons

Do you have a cold/flu or stomach bug? ❑ Yes ❑ No

Stools
See page 5 for scale

Hard   Normal range   Liquid

Comments

95

Day 42

Time	Food and Drink

COMMON ALLERGY TRIGGERS

- ☐ Celery
- ☐ Dairy
- ☐ Eggs
- ☐ Fish
- ☐ Fruit
- ☐ Gluten
- ☐ Lupin(e)
- ☐ Mustard
- ☐ Nuts
- ☐ Sesame Seeds
- ☐ Sulphites
- ☐ Shellfish
- ☐ Soy(a)

96

How are you today?

Time	Symptons

Do you have a cold/flu or stomach bug? ❑ Yes ❑ No

Stools
See page 5 for scale

Hard   Normal range   Liquid

Comments

Day 43

Time	Food and Drink

❑ Celery
❑ Dairy
❑ Eggs
❑ Fish
❑ Fruit
❑ Gluten
❑ Lupin(e)

❑ Mustard
❑ Nuts
❑ Sesame Seeds
❑ Sulphites
❑ Shellfish
❑ Soy(a)

How are you today?

Time	Symptons

Do you have a cold/flu or stomach bug? ❑ Yes ❑ No

Stools
See page 5 for scale

❶ **❷** **❸** **❹** **❺** **❻** **❼**

Hard   Normal range   Liquid

Comments

Day 44

Time	Food and Drink

COMMON ALLERGY TRIGGERS

❑ Celery
❑ Dairy
❑ Eggs
❑ Fish
❑ Fruit
❑ Gluten
❑ Lupin(e)

❑ Mustard
❑ Nuts
❑ Sesame Seeds
❑ Sulphites
❑ Shellfish
❑ Soy(a)

100

How are you today?

Time	Symptons

Do you have a cold/flu or stomach bug? ❑ Yes ❑ No

Stools
See page 5 for scale

❶ ❷ ❸ ❹ ❺ ❻ ❼

Hard   Normal range   Liquid

Comments

Day 45

Time	Food and Drink

COMMON ALLERGY TRIGGERS

❑ Celery
❑ Dairy
❑ Eggs
❑ Fish
❑ Fruit
❑ Gluten
❑ Lupin(e)

❑ Mustard
❑ Nuts
❑ Sesame Seeds
❑ Sulphites
❑ Shellfish
❑ Soy(a)

102

☐ *How are you today?*

Time	Symptons

Do you have a cold/flu or stomach bug? ☐ Yes ☐ No

Stools
See page 5 for scale

Hard   Normal range   Liquid

Comments

Summary table (days 1-23)

Common Triggers	1	2	3	4	5	6	7	8	9	
Any reaction?										
Celery										
Dairy										
Eggs										
Fish										
Fruit										
Gluten										
Lupin(e)										
Mustard										
Nuts										
Sesame Seeds										
Sulphites										
Shellfish										
Soy(a)										
Illness										
Stools (1-7)										
Other										
Other										

How to complete the table

The numbers on the top row are for the days in the diary and the first column shows the common triggers, as well as if your child is

104

	10	11	12	13	14	15	16	17	18	19	20	21	22	23

feeling unwell and if he or she is suffering from less than desirable stools.

Tick all the triggers consumed on the day and place a tick or cross in the *Reaction* row if there is one.

Summary table (days 24-45)

Common Triggers	24	25	26	27	28	29	30	31	32	
Any reaction?										
Celery										
Dairy										
Eggs										
Fish										
Fruit										
Gluten										
Lupin(e)										
Mustard										
Nuts										
Sesame Seeds										
Sulphites										
Shellfish										
Soy(a)										
Illness										
Stools (1-7)										
Other										
Other										

Tick the boxes on the days your child is ill with any sickness so that your results won't be skewed by feeling ill for other reasons than allergies. Their allergies may well be exacerbated by illness as well.

	33	34	35	36	37	38	39	40	41	42	43	44	45

Use the *Bristol Stool Chart* on page 5 to note down your stool health.

The completed table should give a quick overview of days when there are allergic reactions.

MORE BOOKS BY
Ceri Clark

Visit **CeriClark.com** for more information
or buy from **Amazon**

Books for Children

Space Puzzles: Minkie Monster and the Birthday Surprise*
Under the Sea Puzzles: Minkie Monster and the Lost Treasure*
Christmas Puzzles: Minkie Monster Saves Christmas
Children of the Elementi

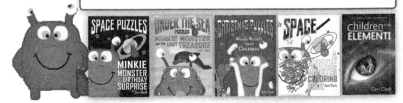

Computer Security Books

Birds Password Book
Bunny Find Your Hoppy Password Book
Meow-nificent Kittens Password Book
Paws-itively Puppies Password Book
A Simpler Guide to Online Security

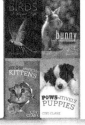
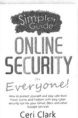

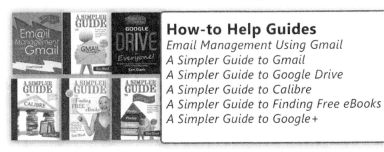

How-to Help Guides

Email Management Using Gmail
A Simpler Guide to Gmail
A Simpler Guide to Google Drive
A Simpler Guide to Calibre
A Simpler Guide to Finding Free eBooks
A Simpler Guide to Google+

Printed by Amazon Italia Logistica S.r.l.
Torrazza Piemonte (TO), Italy

13233085R00069